FOOD and MOOD

Eating Your Way Out of Depression

Erin Stair, MD, MPH

Published by Gray Productions
Guttenberg, New Jersey

Published by Gray Productions
212-315-2449
JudyCorc@aol.com
www.judycorcoran.com

ISBN-10: 153529602x
ISBN-13: 9781535296021
Cover and book design by Judy Corcoran
Printed in August 2016

This book is dedicated to my enchanting, heroic Tara. You were always an inspiration to me and my biggest fan. I never felt worthy, and you never deserved to struggle so much.

While your mental demons were too darn clever, they can never really win or take you away. You remain as strong and beautiful in spirit, and the memory of you is one I'll often visit and always cherish. Thank you for everything.

> *"But I could have told you, Vincent,*
> *the world was never meant*
> *for one as beautiful as you."*
>
> ~ Don McLean, *Vincent*

Contents

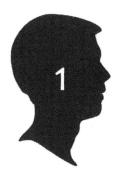

Food Is Mood, Einstein

If you eat crap, you'll feel like crap. It's that simple. If you see a doctor about depression, inattentiveness, anxiety, moodiness, etc., and that doctor does not ask what and how you are eating, get a new doctor. A doctor that doesn't ask about your diet is a bad doctor. I know from a very trying personal experience that depression and generalized moodiness are problems that are sometimes caused by eating unhealthy foods and can be significantly helped and prevented by eating healthy and nutritious foods.

You do not have to be afflicted with a severe eating disorder to have a food problem. Even minor nutrient deficiencies, the wrong diet, or the wrong food ratios can cause you to feel depressed, anxious, tired, moody or irritable. You also need to consider how fast or slowly you are eating, if you are mindful of what you are eating and how much you are eating, if you are eating at the right times, who you are eating with, and whether or not you are eating in a relaxing and healthy environment.

Tweaking your diet so it allows you to feel good and function optimally is an important first step for addressing depression, anxiety or general moodiness, as well as a host of other medical conditions. And trust me—I know this from personal experience. I had a perfectly normal childhood, growing up in rural Pennsylvania, in a town where there were move cows than people, and where I spent a good deal of my time running around. Perhaps that's why I was recruited to play soccer at West Point, the U.S. Military Academy, where

I graduated with a dual degree in chemistry and environmental engineering.

After learning how to kill people, I felt a karmic imbalance. To correct that, I enrolled in Drexel University College of Medicine to learn how to save people. Realizing that people needed to do more for themselves before they ended up with chronic health issues and in the hospital, I went on to earn a Masters of Public Health from New York University's School of Public Health.

Along with all of this, I was bulimic, and I share my bulimia story with you so you can understand why I am so passionate about addressing one's eating habits and lifestyle before recommending he or she take a prescription drug to help with depression or anxiety.

When I was 21, I started over-eating fattening foods and then made myself barf. I am pretty sure I started throwing up to look a little more like Barbie (or was it Skipper?) Or was it because I wanted to be thinner since I thought losing a few pounds would help me run faster on the soccer field? I can't say for sure.

There are many expert theories floating around about bulimia and, as is the case with every psychological disorder, the theories usually connect a disorder's origins to childhood issues. I'm not sure what would happen if you walked into a therapist's office and told him or her that your problem had nothing to do with your childhood, because you had a perfect childhood. They might cry or quit their jobs and join the circus.

Bulimia is not an attractive disease. It's an absolutely disgusting disorder that makes you look bad and feel worse. Your stomach bloats, your breath smells like a corpse is buried under your tongue, your teeth start to look like they've never met a toothbrush, your cheeks swell up like a chipmunk's on steroids, and your knuckles look like they are constantly being attacked by wild beasts. You don't actually end up looking anything like Barbie or Skipper or whomever. I also never ran faster on the soccer field, because, as a bulimic, I was dehydrated, weak and deprived of potassium all of the time.

Besides bulimia's groggy physical effects, you

also feel anxious and depressed. You feel depressed because your body is not getting the right nutrients (if any), and you might also feel depressed about your dwindling cash supply due to spending all of your money on "Food for Vomit." (Instead of "Food for Thought," I referred to my binge purchases as "Food for Vomit.") You may feel depressed because there is a strong addictive component innate to bulimia. Over time, even if you desperately want to stop binging and purging, you can't stop, because you become addicted to the entire maladaptive eating ritual. It really sucks. My entire relationship with food was what the military would call a "Charlie Foxtrot" (CLUSTERF*CK) times infinity.

I remember a psychiatrist telling me that I was depressed because of a lack of serotonin in my brain.

"Erin," he said. "You are depressed. I think we should start you on an antidepressant."

"Oh, I am?" I hadn't connected the dots.

"Yes," he continued. "You have low levels of serotonin in your brain."

"I do? Did you just measure it… telepathically?"

"No," he admitted, taken aback by my biting tone.

"Well then how do you know I'm low in it?"

"Because your answers for the depression questionnaire indicate that you are low in serotonin."

I thought for a moment. "But you didn't measure anything, so how do you know for sure?"

"Well, I don't KNOW for sure," he said, "but I can speculate."

"Now you're changing your story, because before you said I was definitely low in it," I said in an I-gotcha voice.

"Erin, do you want to feel better or not? Am I the expert or are you?" he said, asserting his medical authority. "I can give you a prescription that will correct the problem, but I do not have to."

"Meds?" I said like a teenager.

"Yes, medication."

"Oh, well, yeah. Of course I want meds. Medication is cool."

I went home from that particular doctor's visit with a prescription for an SSRI, which is short for a selective serotonin-reuptake inhibitor. Commonly known as Prozac, Zoloft, Lexapro and Paxil, with prescription on hand, I thought I was a bad-ass. I was still young enough to think having a mental disease was trendy and having medication for my chemically unbalanced brain was cool. Let's face it, once upon a time, being called "crazy" was cool—cool like Angelina Jolie's character in *Girl Interrupted.*

I can also guarantee that on that drive home, I stopped at a grocery store to purchase Food for Vomit, and here's why: The doctor never asked me about my eating habits. If he had asked me, he would have realized that my fatigue, irritability and general moodiness had more to do with the fact that I wasn't allowing my body to absorb the nutrients it needed to run optimally. I puked up everything. I probably puked up serotonin and literally flushed my happiness down the toilet. I didn't have a chemical imbalance or a pill problem. I had a serious food problem, and swallowing a pill was not the answer. Swallowing the right food, and keeping it down, was.

One could argue that the prescribed SSRI would help me overcome my bulimia. But in my case, it never did. My antidepressant made me feel like a zombie with constant dry mouth and no emotions. I was apathetic about everything except my cotton-ball mouth, and I was incapable of fully expressing my emotions, because they felt like they were shoes stuck in gum. I also still binged and purged, so for me, antidepressants were a wash. I remember asking myself every morning, "How is it that a side effect of happy pills is feeling like crap?"

Of course, I had to fix many things in my life to overcome my depression and bulimia. Those things included taming my tendency towards perfection, adopting better sleep habits, learning to be more positive, using humor as a way of healing, finding better social networks, creating a more aggressive exercise routine, and more. All of those things are equally important for overcoming depression or generalized moodiness, but since food is vital for our very survival, I want to focus on that.

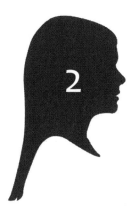

2

Depression 101:
A Quick Look at Some Theories

Unless you are in the medical field, you probably aren't aware of all of the theories of depression. But by reading about them, you will better understand why certain foods help prevent depression and why others can potentially make your depression worse. You will also better understand why I always suggest a diet and lifestyle change over immediately going on antidepressant medication, as long as an individual's circumstances allow for it. Depression is ambiguous and the diagnosis is often subjectively made, and without the assurance of laboratory results, you really have no way of knowing if a certain medication will help you, or if dealing with the medication's side effects is worth it.

Don't stop reading if you are grimacing to yourself right now and saying, "Ugh, science." I promise the following pages will not read like a med-school pathology textbook. I made the explanations quick, truncated, overly simplified, and easy to understand for both nerds and non-nerds. I conducted a focus group with some sixth-graders who told me they understood all of it. (No, not really, but it sounds good.) I promise that Facebook and Pinterest will still be there after you finishing reading this section, so DO NOT skip it.

Also, these are only some of the theories that are known. New ones are constantly being explored, and as time marches on, and if we don't destroy ourselves with nuclear weapons or succumb to global warming, more theories will surely evolve. Which theory is the right one? Maybe one, maybe two, maybe all of them, or maybe none of them. Depression is a multi-factorial illness with biological, social and economic causes. I'm sure factors we haven't even yet considered play a role. It's frustrating.

Will we ever be able to pinpoint the exact cause of depression? Maybe. But I will put the smart money on that answer being a few years (or more) down the road.

1. Where the Spotlight Shines: The Serotonin Hypothesis

The most popular and trendy theory is that a deficiency of serotonin causes depression. Serotonin is a neurotransmitter and neurotransmitters, as the name implies, act as a messenger for neurological information from one cell to another. A serotonin deficiency has been medically linked to depressive symptoms, anxiety and even obsessive-compulsive behaviors.

The low-serotonin theory is a favorite of most drug companies, partly because they have drugs that raise serotonin levels. Therefore, most of the conventional medical treatments for depression are serotonin-reuptake inhibitors (SSRIs), or drugs that increase the amount of serotonin in our brains.

Drug companies heavily market the SSRIs as an effective treatment for depression via TV commercials of medicated people running through fields of colorful flowers, physician endorsements, information pamphlets, pens, scholarly and peer-reviewed journals, and more. All of that marketing has led most people to assume that depression is caused mainly by low levels of serotonin, or what is often recited as a "chemical imbalance in the brain."

You might be saying to yourself, "Well, if that is what is written in a distinguished, peer-reviewed journal, it must be true!" Not so fast, grasshopper. Publication bias is a huge problem with scholarly journals, and drug studies yielding negative results, or results suggesting that the drug is not effective, are about 34% less likely to be published. The drug studies that are published are the ones that have sufficient interest and funding backing them, and therefore, are the ones that dictate modern science.

Also, we would be fools to think that the people

running large drug studies are not at all motivated by the notion of a very large profit if a drug is "statistically-proven" to be effective (Human Nature 101). Therefore, thrifty prevention tools or treatments that do not promise a large monetary return are probably less likely to be studied. (That thought alone is depressing.)

So... is depression really caused by low serotonin? Maybe. Perhaps a proportion of depressed cases are caused by low serotonin. But it is important to understand that no one, as of yet, has measured low levels of serotonin in the brains of depressed people. It is also important to know that a robust body of evidence shows that SSRIs are no better than placebos when treating mild to moderate depression.[1]

That said, I am a HUGE fan of the placebo effect. I mean, why not? If placebos can make us feel better without the downside of side effects, what's the big deal? Well, the big deal with the placebo effect is that its positive effect is only short-term. The placebo effect is a lot like my lucky socks. Whenever I am playing in a soccer game or running a race, I put on this pair of ridiculously bright, multi-colored, knee-high socks. When I am wearing those socks, I am convinced I am a winner. In my head, I become Wonder Woman. However, my lucky-sock effect only lasts for the duration of my soccer game or race. After that, my socks lose their power. (And smell like a rotting corpse). They are no longer lucky...at least not until I wash them for my next big game or race.

If I attempted to wear my lucky socks every day, their brightness would dim, their secret powers would dissipate, and they would eventually become my everyday, boring socks. I would also lose friends, because my lucky socks would smell atrocious. Eventually the dryer will eat my lucky socks, like it does all of my socks, but that's for another book on theories about unsolved sock mysteries.

2. Too Much Stress:
The Glucocorticoid Hypothesis

Have you ever heard someone say, "All this stress is killing me"? Maybe you've even said that. I know I have. Some may call us dramas queen or kings, but there is a lot of truth in that statement. A rapidly expanding body of research is showing the damaging effects that stress has on our bodies, and it is speculated that stress is at the root of 80% of all illnesses. One of those illnesses may be depression.

The Glucocorticoid Cascade Hypothesis is sometimes called HPA (Hypothalamic-Pituitary-Adrenal) Axis Dysregulation, but too many big words, right? In simple terms, HPA Axis Dysregulation means that an individual is dealing with too much stress in his or her life. While short-term spurts of stress may be helpful, chronically high levels of stress are not. For example, if a woman is being chased by a madman with a chainsaw, it is good that she feels stressed and not relaxed. The stress will cause her to run away or fight, whereas no stress would inevitably result in her being hacked into a million little pieces.

Chronic stress, however, is never helpful. It only makes us sick, which is why every person, depressed or not, needs to make time for stress reduction in his or her life. Unfortunately, contemporary lifestyles and mainstream societies are ideal breeding grounds for stress, and therefore, for depression as well.

How do we know for sure that stress leads to depression? We don't know anything for sure. However, researchers have observed that cortisol, the hormone our bodies release during stressful situations, is elevated in depressed patients. In medical terms, Corticotrophin-Releasing Factor (CRF), which stimulates cortisol secretion, is also elevated in depressed patients, and CRF receptors are down-regulated, which is probably due to excessive amounts of CRF.[2,3,4]

We can also tell that stress wreaks havoc on a part of the brain, called the hippocampus, through images. Brain images from patients diagnosed with major depression show atrophy of the hippocampus when compared to brain images of individuals who do not have major depression.[5,6,7]

Why should you care? You should care because it has been shown that chronic stress and excess cortisol can damage this part of the brain and cause it to shrink, which is exactly what the depressed patients' brain images showed. The hippocampus plays a big role in memory, learning and regulating emotions, or more specifically "emotional memories." ("Emotional memory" refers to memories we store because of the emotional impact they had on us.) Under normal conditions, the hippocampus can regulate the HPA axis. An atrophied hippocampus has trouble doing that, which means even more unregulated stress is free to take our bodies and minds as hostages.

Wellness Tip: Meditate, exercise, get a massage, and have hobbies to kill the stress in your life. Think about dancing or floating in a pool. This stuff isn't just "quackerific" hocus pocus. Coping mechanisms can manage stress. Hopefully, your coping mechanisms are peaceful, legal and won't get you arrested or on a "Most Wanted" list. For instance, what if the madman with the chainsaw in my above example was just coping with his stress in a maladaptive way? If only he chose meditation over murder!!! And on that weird note, we'll move on to the next theory.

3. What Becomes of a Broken Heart: The Vascular Hypothesis

This theory for depression mostly applies to

older people who have lived long enough to destroy their arteries by eating all the wrong foods and never exercising. That said, many Americans are eating all the wrong foods, ballooning up and clogging their arteries at younger and younger ages, so perhaps this theory applies to anyone at any age.

Certain risk factors, like eating poorly, not exercising, or having a specific genetic profile, may cause an individual to develop heart or vascular disease. When blood vessels narrow with clogs, you may be in for a heart attack or stroke. Called ischemic heart disease or cerebrovascular disease, both are types of vascular disease. In simple terms, vascular disease means clogged arteries. When your arteries are clogged, blood cannot flow as well. Since blood delivers oxygen and nutrients to our cells, it makes sense why clogged arteries are a problem.

While it is widely accepted that clogged arteries can cause heart attacks and strokes, some researchers speculate that they can lead to depression too.[8] Perhaps vascular disease prevents certain areas of the brain from getting enough oxygen and nourishment. The specific details of the mechanism of action are beyond the scope of this book, but I made up a catchy slogan to remember the Vascular Hypothesis:

When you flow better, you go better!

If you remember that slogan, you'll be happy or happier and go further in life. (I hope. If not, just remember that all sales on this book are final.)

The vascular hypothesis could also be why exercise is PROVEN to help prevent and treat depression, since exercise is also shown to help prevent vascular disease.[9] Yes, exercise causes the release of endorphins, known as the brain's "feel good" chemicals, but it certainly may help fight depression by improving blood flow. I'm a runner, and I run to prevent depression and I know it works. I always tell people that as long as my mile time is faster than my mental demons' times, I am good to go. If someone told me that I couldn't exercise anymore, I guarantee I would get depressed. Let's hope my mental demons don't ever pick up speed. It's also common for an athlete who suffers an injury that prevents doing athletic activity to succumb to temporary depression.

A healthy diet is also proven to help prevent vascular disease, which may also be why it helps prevent depression. Everyone thinks "Eat right and Exercise" is overly simplistic advice, but if everyone actually did it instead of thinking about doing it, we would be a much healthier and happier world.

4. Inflammation-Busters:
The Maladaptive Cytokine Response Theory

This theory is all about inflammation. Inflammation, in a nutshell (no pun intended), is the body's response to a bacteria, virus, allergen, certain foods, a foreign body, or injury. Technically called the Maladaptive Cytokine Response Theory, inflammation is a natural process that allows our bodies to heal from an infection or an injury. So many specialized cells and chemicals take part in an inflammatory response that the immune system resembles an army. Like combat soldiers, the first immune cells on the scene recruit specialized cells with the purpose of either destroying or busting up an invading pathogen (the enemy) or healing an injury (like a military humanitarian mission).

When it comes to destroying an enemy-pathogen, the immune system has a variety of different ways to kill, just like the army does. Many of the immune cells use chemical messengers to communicate with one another. Some of these chemical messengers, called cytokines, travel to the brain to stimulate specific behavioral changes, such as having a reduced appetite, decreased social and physical activity, flattening of mood, feeling pain, impaired learning, fatigue and lack of energy. Do those behavioral changes sound familiar? They sound like what it's like to be sick and what makes you call off from school or work, right?

Even though inflammation is a normal bodily response, it can be part of a disease process such as atherosclerosis (clogging of the arteries), and autoimmune illnesses in which our immune cells attack our own healthy cells (the good guys) instead of the outside invading pathogens (the bad guys). Keeping with the army analogy, immune cells that attack our healthy cells are like tiny Benedict Arnolds. They are complete traitors.

As is the case with stress, too much inflammation (or chronic inflammation) is linked to diseases, including depression. Unfortunately for us, there are many environmental irritants and pathogens that are creating unnecessary inflammation and putting us at a heightened risk for depression and other mental and physical ailments. Man-made pollution and man-made alterations to our environment and food supply have really sabotaged the fight against chronic inflammation. In that sense, we are our own worst enemies.

Let us revisit the technical name and talk about cytokines, or chemical messengers, that play a key part in the immune system. It is already known that specific cytokines, namely Il-1 and TNF-alpha, are involved in the behavioral changes noted above. While these behavioral changes (appetite, mood, fatigue, etc.) are traditionally associated with an acute illness, like a bacterial or viral infection, consider the behavioral changes that occur in depression: fatigue, appetite changes, altered energy metabolism, irritability, etc. One cannot deny that many of those behavioral symptoms overlap with specific behaviors associated with the release of cytokines. Therefore, some scientists theorize that a "maladaptive cytokine response" leads to depression.[10] If an individual has chronically higher levels of cytokines like Il-1 and TNF-alpha, then perhaps he or she is at a heightened risk for depression or depressive-like behavior.

Obviously this theory is hungry for more research. However, it has been shown that when animals are injected with lipopolysaccharide, a molecule that stimulates production of the cytokine Il-1, the animals become depressed.[11]

At the least, definitely remember this theory when people are pushing anti-inflammatory diets of various sorts.

5. When Proteins Go Low:
The BDNF Deficiency Theory

The Brain Derived Neurotrophic Factor Deficiency theory, like the maladaptive cytokine response theory, is also in need of a lot more research. In a nutshell (no pun intended, again), BDNF is a protein that's known to protect nerve cells, enhance neurotransmission, deliver anti-oxidant and anti-depressive activity, and help the brain maintain a normal structure. It probably does even more; we just don't know about it yet. Some studies have shown BDNF to be low in depressed individuals. Other studies have shown that the lower the level of BDNF, the more severe one's level of depression will be.[12,13]

6. Free Radicals Here:
The Oxidative Stress Theory

Oxidative stress occurs when an imbalance exists between the production of reactive oxygen species (free radicals—more bad guys) and their decomposition by antioxidants (more good guys). When we have too much oxidative stress, we have too many free radicals running around and causing damage at multiple sites all over our bodies. While this theory is still in its nadir, it is speculated that oxidative stress can harm the brain and cause depression.[14,15] Everyone can relate to this theory, because I guarantee that everyone, at some point in time, has been told to eat more antioxidants. Or your mother might have yelled, "Eat your vegetables," which is the same thing. This is because antioxidants help our bodies get rid of the dangerous free radicals.

Of course some scientists disagree with this theory entirely. Welcome to science.

7. Insane in the Membrane: The Lipid Bilayer Theory

I will definitely bring up fish oil and omega-three fatty acids later in the book, but a main reason both alternative and conventional doctors tell you to take fish oil to prevent depression is due to the Insane in the Membrane theory. I am really referring to the Lipid Bilayer theory, which I affectionately nicknamed the Insane in the Membrane theory.

This theory is all about cell membranes. All of our cells have a membrane through which nutrients and waste products pass in and out. Sometimes nutrients and waste products do this freely, and other times they must go through a specific channel protein, almost like a toll booth. A well-functioning cell membrane is crucial for our cells to take in the nutrients they need to work right and to kick out all of their waste products. Think of the cell membrane like it's your front door. You want one that works well so the people you want in your house can come in, and the people you want out of your house will get out and stay out. If the door's broken, you might be stuck with people you don't like.

The cell membrane is comprised of a phospholipid bilayer. That means the membrane's top and bottom layers are made up of multiple phosphate heads and long fatty acid tails. To get the picture, think of a row of people standing on their heads. Then think of those people balancing another row of people on their feet so that the two rows of people meet feet to feet. Their heads are the phosphates and their bodies are the fatty acid tails. That, in a nutshell (fine, pun intended), is what a cell membrane looks like.

In regard to depression, I will focus on the fatty acid portion of the cell membrane. Simply put, different kinds of fatty acids can make up a cell membrane, and some fatty acids are more optimal than others. The omega-3 fatty acids (like fish oil) allow the cell membrane to be more flexible and fluid. That means the cell membranes will have an easier time taking in nutrients and getting rid of waste. Omega-6 fatty acids are another story. They make cell membranes more rigid, which makes it more difficult to transport nutrients in and get waste out. Therefore, a diet rich in omega-6 fatty acids, like the standard American diet, can cause cell membranes to function at a less than optimal level, which can then cause brain cells to malfunction and lead to depression.[16,17,18]

Remember my catchy slogan for the vascular hypothesis? "When you flow better, you go better." Well that works for this theory, too.

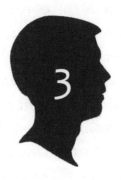

Sad Is Western, Happy Is Mediterranean

The mainstream "Western" diet is made up of mostly processed carbohydrates, fattening and processed meats, chips, white bread, pizza, a ton of sugar, and lots of flavored drinks. It's fast, easy and cheap and anything that is fast, easy and cheap can't be good for you. (I'm sure there's an outlier, but let's not go there.)

The Western diet is linked to a variety of diseases,

including obesity, diabetes, attention deficit disorder, and depression. Most people know it is not the healthiest diet for human beings, yet they still eat it, probably because they become addicted to its convenience and taste. While fast, easy and cheap is never the healthiest option, it is always available, and the globs of fats and processed chemicals make it taste good. Even though it may taste good in the short-term, the Western diet will not make you feel good in the long-term. Here's why:

Sweetened desserts, fried foods, processed meat, refined grains, and high-fat dairy products have all been linked to depression. A 2010 study showed that eating a Western diet increased one's chances of becoming depressed by 38%.[19] A 2007 cross-sectional study showed a lower prevalence of depression in people who ate less fast foods and "ready-to-eat" foods.[20] Another study, the Whitehall II prospective cohort study, also shows that high consumption of sweetened desserts, fried foods, processed meat, high-fat dairy, and refined grains is correlated with higher scores on a particular scale (CES-d) used to screen for depression. Specifically, if one ate such foods, his or her risk for depression increased by 58%.[21]

Another study under the multipurpose Sun Project showed a 40% increased risk for depression in fast food consumers, and a dose-response relationship was observed. A dose-response relationship means that a person's risk of becoming depressed increases proportionally with the amount of fast food he or she eats. Most of the fast food analyzed in this study was pizza, sausage and hamburgers. This study also showed a positive association between the consumption of processed baked goods (muffins, donuts and croissants) and depression, although the observed relationship was not linear and seemed to hit a threshold.[22]

How, exactly, does eating a Western diet make one depressed? Is it as simple as eating crap makes you feel like crap? Maybe. But the previously discussed Vascular Hypothesis, Maladaptive Cytokine Response Theory, Brain Derived Neurotropic Factor Deficiency Theory and Oxidative Stress Theory all may play a role. The Western diet is known to increase the risk of coronary vascular disease, which means the brain may not have optimal blood flow. That could set the stage for depression. The Western diet, and particularly highly refined carbohydrates, is associated with higher amounts of C-reactive Protein, which is an indicator for higher amounts of inflammation in the body and possibly a maladaptive cytokine response.[23,24]

The Western diet is associated with lower amounts of Brain Derived Neurotropic Factor (BDNF) and it also does not contain many antioxidants.[25] Perhaps a higher level of oxidative stress then leads to depression. The truth is no one knows for sure. What can be said is that many studies show that eating a Western diet increases one's risk of becoming depressed.

Eating Our Way Out of Depression

While following the Western diet may mean eating our way into depression, following the Mediterranean diet does the opposite. The essentials of the Mediterranean diet are as follows: eating mostly fruit, vegetables, whole grains and nuts; replacing butter with olive oil; limiting the consumption of red meat to three times per month; and eating fish or chicken twice a week. (While olive oil and nuts are recommended for the Mediterranean diet, and while they both contain the "good kind of fat," I recommend limiting yourself to portioned-out serving sizes. Oils and nuts are extremely calorie dense. Happy AND fat don't often work together, unless you're a dog.)

A recent study published in the *European Journal of Clinical Nutrition* showed that a higher consumption of the Mediterranean diet was associated with a lower prevalence of depression. Another study conducted in Navarra, Spain, and published in the *Archives of General Psychiatry* analyzed 11,000 people for depressive symptoms. The researchers discovered that the risk of becoming depressed was reduced by 30% if the participant followed the Mediterranean diet.

The Mediterranean Diet may help prevent depression because it is associated with less inflammation, less oxidative stress, and improved vascular function. On a personal note, after suffering from depression and having no luck with antidepressants, I put myself on a Mediterranean diet and found that I felt a lot better. Actually, I felt better both physically and mentally. I realize I am only one anecdote, but as the saying goes, "two anecdotes equal data."

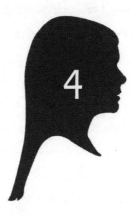

If You Can, Up Your Tryptophan!

Tryptophan is an essential amino acid, which means we cannot manufacture it on our own and need to get it from our diets. It relates to the cause of depression because of its role in serotonin synthesis. Remember the popular Serotonin Hypothesis for depression? It is the hypothesis that suggests low levels of serotonin lead to depression. Tryptophan is a precursor for serotonin. The pathway looks like this:

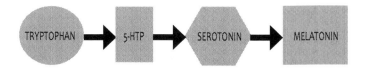

If you extend this pathway out even further, you will see that serotonin is a precursor to melatonin, commonly nicknamed the "Vampire Hormone," because it is the hormone that "only comes out when it's dark" and enables us to get the sleep we need for physical and mental well being. In that sense, melatonin is a good vampire, and one that will help us and not suck us dry.

I am mentioning melatonin, because often times people who are depressed, moody, irritable, etc., do not sleep well. In fact, the relationship between bad sleep and mental illness is a lot like the chicken/egg question. No one has a clue which comes first. The irritable, depressed folks with sleep problems sometimes supplement with melatonin to help them sleep. Perhaps if they ate more tryptophan in their diets (and/or turned off all of the lights and glowing electronics that hinder the release of melatonin), their bodies would naturally synthesize more serotonin and more melatonin, thereby killing two birds with one stone.

Supplement companies make and sell both Tryptophan and 5-HTP capsules for depression. If you walk in any drug store, you will definitely see both products marketed as preventive aids for depression. 5-HTP stands for 5-Hydroxtryptophan, which is another amino acid. While I won't mock anyone who swears by a supplement, I will state my general belief on supplements: The supplement industry is completely unregulated. There is no guarantee you are ingesting EXACTLY what is written on the bottle. Several investigative reports have shown that many supplements do not contain what they claim to contain and sometimes even contain ingredients that we would never want to take.

If you DO want to take a supplement (some people are just "Supplement people"), be sure to really, really, REALLY trust the manufacturer and the seller. Otherwise, you might be pissing away your money on a grandiose marketing pitch. People have been selling snake oil since the beginning of time for a reason: We humans are suckers for a good marketing pitch. The good news is that if you don't want to go the supplement route, you can easily get both tryptophan and 5-HTP from your diet. I'll tell you how in a minute.

While low serotonin is just a hypothesis, there is evidence that acute tryptophan depletion causes depressive symptoms in otherwise healthy individuals.[26,27,28] A review by Reilly et al. even shows that rapid tryptophan depletion can exacerbate both panic and aggression in people.[29] Acute tryptophan depletion is also shown to affect one's ability to learn, which could, arguably, explain a common complaint associated with depression— the inability to concentrate.[30]

A study by Sambeth et al. showed that acute tryptophan depletion impaired both delayed and immediate recall. His study also showed that the impairments were much more severe in females than males.[31] Sambeth's study was especially interesting to me because I suffered from depression during my first two years of medical school, and it really took a toll on my memory. I was always a straight-A student and at the top of my class, yet suddenly I couldn't remember anything I studied. My GPA plummeted to new lows, and I felt useless. I still wonder if I had added more tryptophan to my diet if I would have experienced the same degree of memory impairment. Maybe, maybe not. (That said, there are definitely crazy things I did when I was depressed that I am perfectly happy to forget.)

Another study worth mentioning is one conducted by Robinson et al. He and his gang showed that acute tryptophan depletion causes a negative mood in females who have previously suffered from both depression and acute tryptophan depletion. This could mean that our brain learns to associate "tryptophan depletion" with "bad mood."[32]

The results of Robinson's study also imply that someone who has previously suffered from depression may be at a higher risk for depression if he or she is running low on tryptophan. Many people suffer from a depressive bout, recover and then relapse. Robinson's study is at least one probable theory for that common phenomenon.

Foods High in Tryptophan

chicken breast, roasted
beef tenderloin
turkey
halibut
tuna, yellowfin
shrimp
soybeans, cooked
salmon
milk
cheese

Eat the above foods in moderation and in conjunction with a balanced diet. You don't need to stack your plate with foods high in tryptophan. In fact, you might sabotage yourself if you do that, because tryptophan competes with other amino acids to enter the brain. Your best bet is to eat one of the protein-rich foods listed above along with a baked potato and a side salad. Moderation and balance should always guide ANY and EVERY diet. If they don't, it's a bad diet.

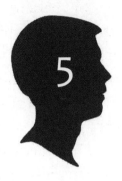

Fish Is Brain Food:
The Omega-3 Fatty Acid Riddle

If you grew up Catholic, like I did, you had to eat fish every Friday. Though I love eating fish now, I hated eating it as a kid. Well, I hated everything if it wasn't pizza, spaghetti or ice cream. To persuade me to eat my fish, my mom would always tell me, "Fish is brain food, Erin!" Back then I thought she meant that I needed to eat fish in order to have a brain.

As my knowledge on the relationship between nutrition and health became a little more sophisticated, I realized I was wrong. You can still have a brain without eating fish. My mom was still right, though. You can have a better brain if you eat fish, and omega-3 fatty acids are the reason why.

Essential omega-3 fatty acids are polyunsaturated fatty acids that come from many plant and marine sources. They are considered "essential" because the human body does not manufacture them naturally, so we have to get them from our diets. Plants are sources of the omega-3 fatty acid, also known as alpha-linolenic acid (ALA), while fish is an excellent source of two preformed omega-3 fatty acids, eicosapentaenoic acid (EPA) and docosahexaenoic acid (DHA).

There are a variety of theories for why omega-3 fatty acids help prevent depression, none of which have been definitively proven. The most prevailing one is that omega-3 fatty acids make cellular membranes more fluid, and thus allow for increased serotonin transport, more effective membrane-imbedded receptor uptake, and better signal transduction.[33,34] Remember when I mentioned, "When you flow better, you go better?" That's what I'm talking about here. Omega-3 fatty acids help form the phospholipid bilayer of cell membranes, which I discussed previously in the section on theories for depression.

Another type of polyunsaturated fatty acids, the omega-6 fatty acids, can also be a part of cell membranes. The omega-6 fatty acids are shown to form much more rigid cell membranes than the omega-3s, which means the membrane may not transfer nutrients and waste as easily. Omega-6 fatty acids are found in corn, safflower, sunflower and soya oils, and they are also precursors to Arachidonic Acid, a molecule that forms our bodies' inflammatory cells, such as leukotrienes, prostaglandins and cytokines.[35] It has been speculated that if an individual eats too many omega-6 fatty acids, he or she may create unnecessary inflammation in his or her body.[36] This "inflammation overload" phenomenon could also relate to the Maladaptive Cytokine Response Theory for depression.

It should not come as a surprise that the Western diet is very high in omega-6 fatty acids and low in omega-3 fatty acids. The Mediterranean diet, which is recommended for depression, is high in omega-3 fatty acids. So even if you forget everything about omega-3 fatty acids, if you remember to follow the Mediterranean diet, you'll be okay. If you prefer to follow an anti-inflammatory diet, also follow the Mediterranean diet. (See how this all comes together?)

A Close Look at Cells

So what are your cell membranes actually made of? The ratio of omega-6 to omega-3 fatty acids that forms the composition of your cell membranes depends on which type of fatty acid you're eating. In short, you're in control. An interesting trend noted by a panel of lipid experts is that the omega-6 intake of Western nations is currently outnumbering the omega-3 intake by a ratio of 15:1.[37] and the recommended ratio is 2:1.[38]

Some experts have correlated this trend with the increasing rate of major depression.[39] It makes sense, considering that depression is now a worldwide epidemic when at the same time more and more people all over the globe are eating a Western diet.

Weissman et al. conducted a study that included a great graph that I love to share when talking about omega fatty acids and depression. He and his team conducted a large, cross-national comparison between the prevalence of major depression and fish consumption. The results of his study, which included 35,000 participants, are rooted in an extremely reliable, cross-national database. His study shows a statistically significant negative association between national rates of major depression and fish consumption. This means that as the consumption of fish goes down in a country, the rate of depression goes up. New Zealand had the highest rate of depression and the lowest fish consumption, while Japan had the highest fish consumption and lowest rate of major depression.[40] Since nothing says it better than a picture, take a look on the graph on the next page.

An earlier study by Maes and his team showed

Prevalence of major depression and fish consumption

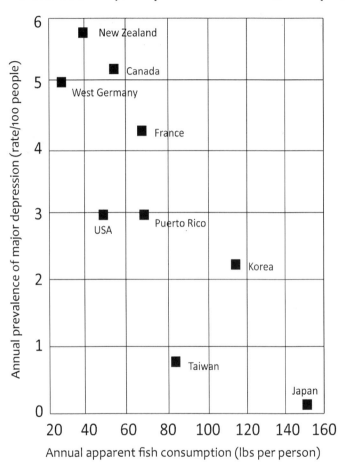

a lower concentration of omega-3 fatty acids in depressed patients compared to those who were not depressed, and a significant increase in the ratio of Arachidonic Acid to EPA.[41]

Another early study by Edwards showed that the red blood cell membranes of depressed patients had significantly lower levels of omega-3s compared to healthy people, and a significant positive correlation between dietary intake of omega-3 fatty acids and the concentration of omega-3 fatty acids in red blood cell membranes.[42] His study provides some evidence that we can control the health of our cell membranes with our diet!

McNamara and his team measured levels of DHA (docosahexaenoic acid) in the postmortem brains of patients diagnosed with major depression and compared them to brains of people who were not depressed. He found significantly lower levels of DHA in the patients who had been diagnosed with depression, and interestingly enough, a 32% deficiency in depressed females compared to a 16% deficiency in depressed males.[43]

In addition to the "Insane in the Membrane"

Theory for depression, a deficiency in omega-3 fatty acids has also been linked to the Vascular Hypothesis for depression. To review, the Vascular Hypothesis is that the brain is not receiving optimal blood flow due to clogged or deficient arteries, which then sets the stage for depression. Several studies have shown that coronary artery disease (clogged arteries) correlates with low levels of omega-3 fatty acids.[44,45,46] The take-home point is that eating omega-3 fatty acids may very well help blood flow better to your heart and your brain, therefore improving both your heart and brain function.

Omega-3 fatty acids may also be related to the Glucocorticoid Cascade (too much stress) Hypothesis. I already mentioned that depressed people have higher levels of cortisol.[47] Studies on animals have shown that high levels of cortisol, the major stress hormone, can deactivate liver enzymes that transform short fatty acids into the longer-chained omega-3 fatty acids.[48] Of course the relationship between chronic stress and depression is a lot like the relationship between poor sleep and depression and a lot like the relationship between

~ 53 ~

the chicken and the egg. It is impossible to know which one came first. All we know is that they are definitely related.

An interesting study by Delarue and his team showed that blood cortisol levels were significantly lowered when individuals supplemented with 7.2 grams/day of omega-3 fish oil.[49,50] Does this mean loading our diets with omega-3 fatty acids is the secret to beating chronic stress, depression, and all of the other illnesses associated with chronic stress? No, not at all. But it certainly can't hurt.

Omega-3 fatty acids may even relate to the Brain-derived Neurotrophic Factor (BDNF) Deficiency Theory for depression. As mentioned before, BDNF is shown to be lower in depressed patients. A 2004 study conducted on rats at the University of California, Los Angeles, showed that omega-3 fatty acids can increase the production of BDNF, while a diet high in sugars and saturated fats inhibit its production.[51] What diet is high in sugar and fats? The Western diet! So again, when it comes to diet, go Mediterranean and ditch the West.

While a deficiency of omega-3 fatty acids may

lead to depression, does eating omega-3 fatty acids help prevent depression? Maybe. Some studies say yes and others say no.

One study conducted by the University of Navarra in collaboration with the Harvard School of Public Health showed that a moderate consumption of fish (between 83.3-112g/day) resulted in a 30% reduced chance of developing major depression.[52] An interesting finding in this study is that participants who had a very high baseline consumption of omega-3 fatty acids and subsequently increased their consumption during the study, actually developed an increased risk for mental illness. Some of the researchers involved with the study speculated that this unexpected trend was due to high mercury content in the consumed fish, since mercury is known to cause neurological damage and mental problems.[53]

It is important to keep in mind that some fish contain high levels of mercury and other toxins. This problem will only get worse as our oceans become more and more polluted, which is another reason you should always practice moderation in your diet.

In other words, eat fish for the benefits of omega-3 fatty acids, but don't eat so much fish that you put yourself at risk for mercury poisoning. The toxicity is in the dose!

A study by Rizzo and his team showed that fish oil supplements significantly improved depressive symptoms in depressed patients while supplementing with placebo pills did not.[54] Su and his research team conducted a similar study to Rizzo and also showed that fish oil supplements significantly improved depressive symptoms.[55]

If you are already taking antidepressants for depression, you may want to also consider eating more omega-3fatty acids. A study by Nemets and his team showed that adding omega-3 fatty acids via fish oil capsules to concurrent antidepressant therapy significantly improved treatment results.[56]

Though I am a bigger fan of getting nutrients from food over supplements, if you decide to supplement with omega-3 fatty acids, the ratio of EPA to DHA seems to matter. In most of the studies that yielded positive results for omega-3 fatty acid supplements and depression, an EPA to DHA ratio of approximately 2:1 was used. It is speculated that the EPA content is the main driver of the effects omega-3 fatty acids have on depression, and some experts even suggest using only pure EPA.[57,58,59]

Some omega-3 researchers suggest that all fish oil protocols contain at least 60% of EPA for maximum effectiveness.[60] That percentage is something to keep in mind if you purchase an omega-3 fatty acid supplement. The supplement market is saturated with omega-3 fatty acid potions and pills of all sorts of ingredients and ratios. A good lot of them don't work, so again, if you want to go the supplement route, do your homework and find a manufacturer you know you can trust. You want an optimal fish oil not a fraudulent snake oil.

Foods High in Omega-3 Fatty Acids

Vegetarian
flaxseed
walnuts
hemp
leafy vegetables
(kale and spinach)
pumpkin seeds
mint
fortified foods

Animal
salmon
herring
mackerel
trout
sardines
tuna
halibut

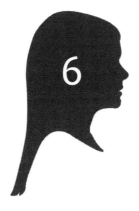

Fill Your Plate with Magnesium-Rich Goodies!

The element magnesium is utilized by every cell in our bodies and is needed for a variety of cellular processes to function properly. A magnesium deficiency has been linked to a laundry list of physical and mental ailments, including depression. Jacka and his team of researchers analyzed the relationship between dietary magnesium intake and depression in 5,708 participants as part of the Hordaland Health

Study. They found that a low magnesium intake was linked to higher levels of depression.[61]

The link between low levels of magnesium and depression remained statistically significant even after the research team controlled for all potential confounding factors. Jacka also analyzed the relationship between low magnesium intake and anxiety, but that correlation did not prove significant.

Another study by Iosifescu and his team involved brain imaging to show that there were decreased levels of intracellular magnesium in the brains of individuals diagnosed with treatment-resistant depression.[61]

A very intriguing relationship is the one between magnesium and attempted suicide. If it isn't obvious, depressed people may attempt suicide. Banki and his team of researchers measured magnesium levels in the cerebrospinal fluid (CSF) of 41 psychiatric patients and compared them to non-psychiatric patients. They discovered that magnesium levels were significantly lower in individuals who attempted suicide.[62] A similar study by Levine and his team measured magnesium levels in the CSF of extremely depressed patients who were just admitted to the hospital.[63] Results of Levine's study showed that magnesium levels were significantly lowered in the CSF of these patients. I should also note that calcium levels were elevated in these patients. Both high calcium and low magnesium have been associated with depression.[64]

Low magnesium may be linked to the Oxidative Stress Theory for depression, the one about free radicals that we discussed earlier. Several studies have shown that consuming a diet low in magnesium leads to increased oxidative stress in both plasma and tissues.[65,66]

Another theory is that a magnesium deficiency alters an individual's energy metabolism and therefore leads to symptoms of depression. Some animal studies and post-mortem samples from depressed individuals have shown that low magnesium correlates to lower amounts of the enzyme Glutamate Dehydrogenase (GDH1).[67,68,69] GDH1 is an important enzyme involved in the tricarboxcylic acid cycle, or essentially, ATP production (adenosine triphosphate, coenzyme used as an energy carrier in the cells of all known organisms). Of course ATP is our body's key energy molecule, so it makes sense that interfering with its production could make someone feel below par.

Another theory is that a diet low in magnesium leads to an over-activation of an enzyme, NO synthase, which leads to too much Nitric Oxide in the brain. Too much Nitric Oxide has been associated with a myriad of mental problems, including symptoms of depression.[70,71]

Does supplementing with magnesium work as well as medication for depression? Maybe. It surely depends on the cause of an individual's depression, as well as his or her current magnesium level and biochemical profile. Still, a really interesting study was conducted by Barragan-Rodriguez and friends. They did a randomized controlled trial in which depressed patients with low magnesium were either treated with magnesium or treated with Imipramine, a tricylic antidepressant drug. They discovered that supplementing with magnesium was as effective for treating depression as the drug Imipramine.[72]

Though I am skeptical of oral supplements, here is an example in which they proved successful. That said, the magnesium levels of all of the patients were measured and proven to be low beforehand, and the supplement was deemed safe, as well as part of a controlled experiment.

Ladies who suffer from mood swings or depression as part of PMS or premenstrual syndrome (and those brave souls who have to do deal with us), should consider eating more magnesium in their diets. A lot of research has suggested a magnesium deficiency in women who suffer from PMS, and even more importantly, several studies have shown that magnesium significantly helps alleviate mood swings, depression and even the fluid retention and bloating commonly associated with PMS.[73,74,75,76]

On a personal note, I know that my moodiness gets much worse when I have PMS. My historical bouts of PMS have caused me a lot of dysfunction, including unnecessary fighting with family, friends and strangers in grocery lines, impulsively quitting jobs and schools like I just won the lottery (when in fact, I did not win the lottery), ridiculously high consumption of alcohol which made me act stupidly, and I've lost quite a few boyfriends who ran for the hills during that time. So, trust me when I say that I now eat a lot of magnesium the week before "my friend" comes to town.

Foods Rich in Magnesium

sesame seeds
dill
pine nuts
almonds
spearment
Brazil nuts
chocolate
sunflower seeds
basil
broccoli
okra
spinach
watermelon seeds
chives

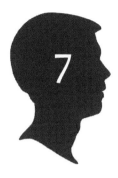

The Importance of B12 and Folate!

If you are feeling moody or depressed or both, you may need to increase the amount of folate and B12 in your diet. B12 is a water-soluble vitamin that has many important functions in the body, including the formation of red blood cells and the maintenance of healthy nerves. Folate (and Folic Acid) is a form of the water-soluble B vitamin. Since the mid-1940s, doctors and researchers have observed that deficiencies in either folate or B12 result in behavioral, psychological and neural complications.[77]

The most important reason for discussing folate and B12 together is that they are both involved in the metabolism of the amino acid homocysteine to methionine. High levels of homocysteine are not only directly toxic to nerve cells, but have also been linked to depression, schizophrenia, Alzheimer's disease and Parkinson's disease.[78] The take-home point is this: If you have low levels of either B12 or folate, you put yourself at a higher risk of not being able to effectively metabolize homocysteine and therefore having dangerously high levels of it in your body. A higher level of homocysteine means you have a higher risk of developing neural and/or mental problems.

Vitamin B12 is also a necessary cofactor for making SAM-e, a molecule that serves as the brain's major methyl donor. SAM-e has also been shown to have antidepressant effects.[79] You might recognize SAM-e from the drug store, since many companies make it and sell it as a "natural" cure for depression. Does the SAM-e supplement work? Your guess is as good as mine. Without regulation over the supplement industry, we have no way of knowing what exactly is in a bottle labeled "SAM-e" or how effective it is. Therefore, I would strongly recommend trying to increase levels of SAM-e naturally by getting more B12 in your diet.

There are a lot of studies showing that low levels of B12 are associated with higher rates of depression. For example, Penninx and friends conducted a study on 700 community-bound women showing that those participants with a B12 deficiency were two times more likely to be severely depressed.[80] A more recent study involving 199 depressed patients showed that supplementing with Vitamin B12 can significantly improve depressive symptoms.[81]

Research has shown that depressed patients have lower concentrations of folate than people who are not depressed.[82,83,84] It has also been shown that a folate deficiency is associated with a more severe bout of depression.[85] Another study concluded that supplementing with 15mg of L-methyfolate a day is an effective treatment strategy for individuals with a major depressive disorder who experience no response to SSRIs.[86] This finding is encouraging considering that SSRIs are the most common drugs prescribed for depression, and many people do not respond to them.

Foods High in B12

beef	calf's liver
venison	lamb
salmon	shrimp
halibut	scallops

Foods High in Folate

fortified cereals	spinach
cooked lentils	eggs
brussels sprouts	broccoli
asparagus	cantaloupe
avocado	okra

folate-enriched pasta
Great Northern beans

Vitamin E and Selenium

Vitamin E is best known for its antioxidant properties and its role in preventing heart disease and some types of cancer. Of course, taking too much Vitamin E has been associated with negative health effects, so the key here is balance. Some research has shown that a low Vitamin E level is linked to major depression. A 2004 study showed that plasma levels of Vitamin E, called Tocopherol, were significantly lower in patients diagnosed with major depression.[87] This study also showed that plasma levels of Vitamin E were inversely related to people's scores on a standardized test, the Beck Depression Inventory, used to diagnose depression. Of course, causation cannot be proven in the above cross-sectional study, so it is hard to determine whether low Vitamin E causes depression or vice versa.

Another study by Maes and pals showed that Vitamin E levels were significantly lower in majorly depressed patients compared to healthy volunteers. It is speculated that lower levels of Vitamin E lowers one's antioxidant potential and that is why depressed individuals are at a heightened risk for other illnesses.[88]

The association between Vitamin E and depression is not always clear and requires a lot more research. For example, The Rotterdam Study, which evaluated 3,884 adults over 60 years of age, did not find a significant association between Vitamin E levels and major depression once biological, nutritional and social factors were taken into consideration.[89] Conflicting study results like these (more common than not in science), are good reasons to never overdo or underdo anything. Always strive for balance. In simple words, make sure you are getting enough Vitamin E in your diet, and don't eat too much or too little. Moderation is always a safe approach.

The element Selenium has also been linked to depression. A study by Finely and Penland showed that a high intake of dietary selenium improved mood and one's confidence level and reduced anxiety, whereas a diet low in selenium increased feelings of depression and hostility.[90] Heck, if you are sad AND angry (and an ax is conveniently nearby), try leaving the ax alone and going out for a selenium-rich meal.

Another study by Benton and Cook showed that supplementing with 100 mcg (micrograms) of selenium on a daily basis for five weeks resulted in an elevation of mood as well as a decrease in anxiety.[91] The same study showed that lower levels of selenium in the diet correlated with more reports of depression, anxiety and fatigue.[92]

There are several theories as to why low selenium could cause depression. Selenium is required to synthesize thyroid hormone, and low thyroid hormone (or being hypothyroid) is associated with depression, fatigue and sluggishness. A selenium deficiency may reduce the ability of the body's immune system to function optimally. Selenium is also an essential component of an important antioxidant enzyme, so it is possible that a low level of selenium increases oxidative stress and predisposes an individual to depression. All of these theories are pure speculation. The only certainty is that we should attempt to get a healthy amount of selenium in our diets.

Foods High in Vitamin E

wheat germ   sunflower oil
safflower oil   soybean oil
broccoli   kiwi
almonds   peanut butter
hazel nuts, dry roasted   mango
sunflower seeds, kernels, dry roasted
spinach, frozen chopped boiled
corn oil (salad or vegetable oil)

Foods Rich in Selenium

tuna   chicken breast
cod   whole eggs
beef   turkey
oatmeal, instant fortified cooked
Brazil nuts, dried unblanched
low-fat cottage cheese
enriched noodles

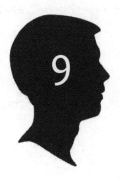

Warding Off Depressing
Demons with Good Food

This book started by looking at the connection between what you eat and how you feel. Trust me, it's real. Just eat 16 bags of Cheetos some night and see how you feel the next day. Or rent the film, *Supersize Me*, about a man who ate three meals a day at McDonald's for a month.

We then looked at the many theories of depression, and there are many. Depression doesn't just come from a bad breakup, financial worries, or a job loss. There are medical and chemical issues at play. A serotonin deficiency tops the list and is followed by how the body reacts chemically to too much stress and how clogged vascular arteries and too much inflammation in the arteries prevent good health. I also talked about chemical imbalances including a deficiency of the BDNF protein, too many free radicals, and cell membranes that don't function well. All of these can lead to depression.

What's the quick fix? One thing that will make a huge difference in your level of depression is your diet. Switching to a Mediterranean-based diet will make you healthier than almost anything else you can do. And what's the diet's secret? The key components are:

- Eating plant-based foods, such as fruits, vegetables, whole grains, legumes and nuts
- Replacing unhealthy fats such as butter with healthy fats such as olive and canola oil
- Flavoring your food with spices and herbs rather than salt
- Limiting red meat to a few times a month

- Eating fish and poultry at least twice a week
- Drinking wine in moderation

What else helps lift your depression? Tryptophan, omega-3 fatty acids, magnesium-rich foods, Vitamin B12 and folate, and Vitamin E and Selenium. I've already listed foods that are rich in these acids and vitamins, but think plant-based fruits and vegetables, whole grains, legumes, nuts, fish, poultry and lean meat occasionally. Ha! Just like the Mediterranean Diet. And did you notice what's missing? Sugar! Read on.

The Sugar Riddle

In addition to a sugar high, like when a child eats too many cookies and starts bouncing off the walls, sugar can cause a sugar low. Sugar levels that spike and crash throughout the day create feelings of depression, moodiness, tiredness and just a generalized feeling of BLAH. If your sugar is crashing and burning throughout the day, so will your brain. You need to work on maintaining a balanced relationship with sugar.

To avoid the sugar highs and lows, you can try doing what I do and eat foods that have low glycemic loads. A food's glycemic load is determined by how much its carbohydrate amount raises the blood glucose (sugar) level. It is more accurate than the "glycemic index," because it takes into account the amount of carbohydrates present in one serving size.

A Few Big Tips: Start a Food Diary

Whenever I start working with a wellness client, the first thing I make him or her do is start a food diary. A food diary should at least include what you're eating, when you're eating, how you feel when you eat, who you're eating with, and the environment in which you're eating. No matter what your personal wellness goals may be, a food diary is crucial.

Most people think keeping a food diary is only helpful if you want to lose weight. Not so. It can help you evaluate unhealthy eating patterns, yes, but it can also help you identify if you're allergic to a specific food; if certain foods are making your stomach sick or giving you indigestion; if certain foods are making you feel tired or moody; if you aren't following a good feeding schedule; if you are eating in a stressful environment; how the people you often eat with make you feel; how you feel when you eat, and more.

The point is that if you physically do not feel good when you're eating or after you eat, your mood will also suffer. No one feels good if they constantly have an irritable bowel or stomach pains after eating. A food diary can help you see patterns and make beneficial changes that will optimize your eating habits and eating environment, all of which will naturally help boost your mood.

Look Closely at Alcohol

There's nothing wrong with cracking a beer or pouring a glass of wine after a long day or with your meal. But know that alcohol, metabolically, is a depressant, and if you are fighting depression or looking to improve your moods, take a close look at how much alcohol you drink, how often, and how you feel the next day.

Exercise

No one needs to hear again that daily exercise is important to your overall health. But if you're not moving around, and if you find that sifting through remote controls, trying to find the one for Netflix, is taking up a good part of your time, you may want to consider taking some sort of action. In opposition to alcohol, exercise and activity produce endorphins, which are actually mood enhancers. And if you ever want to feel better immediately, just put on some music and dance. An Australian study published in the journal, *Music and Medicine*, showed that dancing the tango has significant health benefits for people experiencing mood disorders.[95]

The authors wrote that participants showed significant reductions in depression, anxiety, stress, and insomnia. So try killing two birds with one stone! Turn up the radio and dance your depression away. Or pop in some ear buds and go for a walk. Communing with Mother Nature can do wonders for depression, too.

Eat with Family and Friends

There's a reason families and friends eat together. Humans are social creatures and from the start of time have broken bread and shared meals together. If you find yourself alone in front of the TV for most meals, make a plan to eat with others. Even going to a local restaurant where you become a "regular" can improve your eating habits and mood.

No matter how good a cook you are, your food will taste better if you set a nice table. If you're eating off of paper plates amid empty pizza boxes and Chinese food cartons, tidy up a little before your meal. Scoop that rice or pizza onto a nice plate and use a real fork. Your surroundings are part of your life and you have the ability to enjoy them.

Learn to Be Thankful While You Are Eating

Many studies in the realm of positive psychology have shown that having a sense of gratitude correlates with less depressive symptoms.[93,94] In fact, traditional psychiatrists are prescribing Positive Activity Interventions (PAIs) to depressed patients, and one of these is making a daily list of things you are grateful for. So why not make mealtime a PAI? It can be as simple as taking a minute to think about how grateful you are for the food in front of you, especially in a world where so many go without. If you are religious, this type of PAI is similar to saying grace, but you certainly do not have to be religious to feel thankful for food in front of you. Expressing gratitude is free, has no negative side effects, and is something you can do anywhere. Give it a shot. You might surprise yourself by how good it makes you feel.

Going Forward

I hope the many theories and suggestions in this book are helpful to you. If you're battling depression, there could be many causes and many remedies. The most important thing, however, is to seek help and know that you are not alone.

Bibliography

1 Fournier, J. et al. (2010). Antidepressant Drug Effects and Depression Severity. JAMA, 303(1).

2 Herbert, J. (2013). Cortisol and depression: three questions for psychiatry. Psychological Medicine, 43(3).

3Cowen, P. J. (2002). Cortisol, serotonin, and depression: all stressed out? The British Journal of Psychiatry, 180.

4 Hauger, R., et al. (2009). Role of CRF receptor signaling in stress vulnerability, anxiety, and depression. Annals of the New York Academy of Sciences, 117.

5 Nestler, E. J., et al. (2002). Neurobiology of depression. Neuron, 34.

6 Stahl, S. M., et al. (2008). The potential role of a corticotrophin-releasing factor receptor-1 antagonist in psychiatric disorders. CNS Spectrums, 13(6).

7 Bremner, J. D., et al. (2002). Structural changes in the brain in depression and relationship to symptom recurrence. CNS Spectrums, 7 (2).

8Sneed, J. R., et al. (2011). The vascular depression hypothesis: an update. American Journal of Geriatric Psychiatry, 19(2).

9 Mammen, G., et al. (2013). Physical Activity and the prevention of depression: a systematic review of prospective studies. American Journal of Preventive Medicine, 45(5).

Bibliography

10 Dantzer, R., et al. (2008). From inflammation to sickness and depression: when the immune system subjugates the brain. Nature Reviews Neuroscience, 9.

11 Bison, S., et al. (2009). Differential behavioral, physiological, and hormonal sensitivity to LPS challenge in rats. International Journal of Interferon, Cytokine, and Mediator Research.

12 Shimizu, E., et al. (2003). Alternations of serum levels of brain-derived neurotrophic factor (BDNF) in depressed patients with or without antidepressant. Biological Psychiatry,54(1).

13 Karege, F., et al. (2002). Decreased serum brain-derived neuro-trophic factor levels in major depressed patients. Psychiatry Research 109(2).

14 Michel, T. M. (2012). The role of oxidative stress in depressive disorders. Current pharmaceutical design, 18(36).

15 Chung, C. P., et al. (2013). Increased oxidative stress in patients with depression and its relationship to treatment. Psychiatry Research, 206.

16 Sanchez-Villegas, A., et al. (2007). Long chain omega-3 fatty acid intake, fish consumption and mental disorders in the SUN cohort study. European Journal of Nutrition, 46, 337-346.

17 Logan, A. (2006). Omega-3 Fatty Acids and depression. Positive Health, 24-29.

18 Rizzo, A., et al. (2012). Comparison between the AA/EPA ratio in depressed and non-depressed elderly females: omega-three fatty acid supplementation correlates with improved symptoms but does not change immunological parameters. Nutrition Journal, 11(82).

19 Jacka, F., et al. (2010). Association of western and traditional diets with depression and anxiety in women. American Journal of Psychiatry, 167.

20 Liu, C., et al. (2007). Perceived stress, depression and food consumption frequency in the college students of China Seven Cities. Physiology & Behavior, 92(4).

21 Akbaraly, T., et al. (2009). Dietary pattern and depressive symptoms in middle age. The British Journal of Psychiatry, 195(5).

22 Sanchez-Villegas, A., et al. (2011). Fast-food and commercial baked goods consumption and the risk of depression. Public Health Nutrition, 15(3).

23 Mente, A., et al. (2009). A systematic review of the evidence supporting a causal link between dietary factors and coronary heart disease. Archives of Internal Medicine, 169(7).

24Yunsheng, M., et al. (2006). Association between dietary fiber and serum C-reactive protein. The American Journal of Clinical Nutrition, 83(4).
25Numakawa, T., et al. (2014). The role of brain-derived neurotrophic factor in comorbid depression: possible linkage with steroid hormones, cytokines, and nutrition. Front Psychiatry, 5(136).

26 Ardis, T. C., et al. (2009). Effect of acute tryptophan depletion on noradrenaline and dopamine in the rat brain. Journal of psychopharmacology, 23(1).

27 Evers, E. A., et al. (2010). The effects of acute tryptophan depletion on brain activation during cognition and emotional processing in healthy volunteers. Current Pharmaceutical Design, 16(18).

Bibliography

28 Reilly, J. G., et al. (1997). Rapid depletion of plasma tryptophan: a review of studies and experimental methodology. Journal of psychopharmacology, 11(4).

29 Ibid

30 Evers, E. A., et al. (2005). Serotonergic modulation of prefrontal cortex during negative feedback in probabilistic reversal learning. Neuropsychopharmacology, 30(6).

31 Sambeth, A., et al. (2007). Sex differences in the effect of acute tryptophan depletion on declarative episodic memory: a pooled analysis of nine studies. Neuroscience and biobehavioral reviews, 31(4).

32 Robinson, O. J., et al. (2009). Acute tryptophan depletion evokes negative mood in healthy females who have previously experienced concurrent negative mood and tryptophan depletion. Psychopharmacology, 205(2).

33 Sanchez-Villegas, A., et al. (2007). Long Chain Omega-3 Fatty Acid Intake, Fish Consumption and Mental Disorders in the SUN Cohort Study. European Journal of Nutrition, 46, 337-346.

34 Edwards, R., et al. (1998). Omega-3 polyunsaturated fatty acid levels in the diet and in red blood cell membranes of depressed patients. Journal of Affective Disorders, 48.

35 Rizzo, A., et al. (2012). Comparison between the AA/EPA ratio in depressed and non-depressed elderly females: omega-three fatty acid supplementation correlates with improved symptoms but does not change immunological parameters. Nutrition Journal, 11(82).

36 Simopoulos, A. P. (2013). The importance of the ratio of omega-6/omega-3 essential fatty acids. Biomedicine & Pharmacotherapy, 56 (8).

37 Simopoulos, A. P. (2008). The importance of the Omega-6/Omega-3 fatty acid ratio in cardiovascular disease and other chronic diseases. Experimental Biology and Medicine, 223(6).

38 Simopoulos, A. P., Leaf, A. & Salem, N.(1999). Workshop on the Essentiality of and Recommended Dietary Intakes for Omega-6 and Omega-3 Fatty Acids. Journal of the American College of Nutrition, 18.

39 Weissman M., Bland, R. & Canino, G.(1996). Cross-national Epidemiology of Major Depression and Bipolar Disorder. JAMA (276), 293-299.

40Ibid.

41 Maes, M., Smith, R., Christophe, A., Cosyns, P., Desnyder, R. & Mettzer, H. (1996). Fatty Acid Composition in Major Depression Decreased with Fractions in Cholesteryl Esters and Increased C20: 4w6/C20:5w3 Ratio in Cholesteryl Esters and Phospholipids. Journal of Affective Disorders, 38, 35-46.

42 Edwards, R., et al. (1998). Omega-3 polyunsaturated fatty acid levels in the diet and in red blood cell membranes of depressed patients. Journal of Affective Disorders, 48.

43 McNamara, R., Hahn, C & Jandacek, R. (2007). Selective deficits in the omega-3 fatty acid docosahexaenoic acid in postmortem orbitofrontal cortex of patients with major depressive disorder. Biological Psychiatry, 62 (1), 17-24.

44 Kris-Etherton, P., Harris, W., & Appel, L. (2003). Fish Consumption, Fish Oil, Omega-3 Fatty Acids, and Cardiovascular Disease. Arteriosclerosis, Thrombosis and Vascular Biology, 23.

Bibliography

45 Leaf, A., Kang, J., Xiao, Y., & Billman, G. (2003). Clinical Prevention of Cardiac Death by n-3 Polyunsaturated Fatty Acids and Mechanism of Prevention of Arrhythmias by n-3 Fish Oils. Circulation 107.

46 Frasure-Smith, N., Lesperance, F., & Pierre, J. (2004). Major Depression Is Associated with Lower Omega-3 Fatty Acid Levels in Patients with Recent Acute Coronary Syndromes. Biological Psychiatry, 55.

47 Dziurkowska, E., Wesolowski, M., Dziurkowski, M. (2013). Salivary Cortisol in Women with Major Depressive Disorder Under Selective Serotonin Reuptake Inhibitors Therapy. Archives of Women's Mental Health,16(2),139-147.

48 Frasure-Smith, N., Lesperance, F., & Pierre, J. (2004). Major Depression Is Associated with Lower Omega-3 Fatty Acid Levels in Patients with Recent Acute Coronary Syndromes. Biological Psychiatry, 55.

49 Delarue, J., Matzinger, O., Binnert, C., Schneiter, P., Chiolero, R. & Tappy, L. (2003). Fish Oil Prevents the Adrenal Activation Elicited by Mental Stress in Healthy Men. Diabetes & Metabolism, 29(3), 289-95.

50 Kempton, M., Salvador, Z., Munafo, M., Geddes, J., Simmons, A., Frangou, S. & Willams, S. (2011). Structural Neuroimaging Studies in Major Depressive Disorder: Meta-Analysis and Comparison with Bipolar Disorder. Jama, 68(7).

51 Wu, A., Zhe, Y. & Fernando, G. Dietary Omega-3 Fatty Acids Normalize BDNF Levels, Reduce Oxidative Damage, and Counteract Learning Disability after Traumatic Brain Injury in Rats. Journal of Neurotrauma, 21(10).

52 Sanchez-Villegas, A., Henriquez, P., Figueiras, A., Ortuno, F., La-
hortiga, F. & Martinez-Gonzalez, M. (2007). Long Chain Omega-3
Fatty Acid Intake, Fish Consumption and Mental Disorders in the
SUN Cohort Study. European Journal of Nutrition, 46.

53Ibid.

54 Rizzo, A., Corsetto, P., Montorfano, G., Opizzi, A., Faliva, M., Gia-
cosa, A. & Rondanelli, M. (2012). Comparison between the AA/EPA
ratio in depressed and non-depressed elderly females: omega-3 fatty
acid supplementation correlates with improved symptoms but does not
change immunological parameters. Nutrition Journal, 11(82).

55 Su, K.P., Huang, S., Chiu, C.,& Shen, W. (2003). Omega-3 Fatty
Acids in Major Depressive Disorder: A Preliminary Double-Blind,
Placebo-Controlled Trial. European Journal of Neuropsychophar-
macology, 13.

56 Nemets, B., Stahl, Z., & Belmaker, R. H. (2002). Addition of
Omega-3 Fatty Acid to Maintenance Medication Treatment for
Recurrent Unipolar Depressive Disorder. The American Journal of
Psychiatry, 159.

57 Martins, J.G., Bensten, H. & Puri, B.K. (2012). Eicosapentaenoic
Acid Appears to be the Key Omega-3 Fatty Acid Component Associated with Efficacy in Major Depressive Disorder: A Critique of Bloch
and Hannestad and Updated Meta-Analysis. Molecular Psychiatry.

58 Puri, B. K. (2001). Eicosapentaenoic Acid in Treatment-Resistant
Depression Associated with Symptom Remission, Structural Brain
Changes and Reduced Neuronal Phospholipid Turnover. Interna-
tional Journal of Clinical Practice, 55.

Bibliography

59 Horrobin, D.F. (2002). A New Category of Psychotropic Drugs: Neuroactive Lipids as Exemplified by Ethyl Eicosapentaenoate. Progress in Drug Research (59).

60 Martins, J.G., Bensten, H. & Puri, B. K. (2012). Eicosapentaenoic Acid Appears to be the Key Omega-3 Fatty Acid Component Associated with Efficacy in Major Depressive Disorder: A Critique of Bloch and Hannestad and Updated Meta-Analysis. Molecular Psychiatry.

61 Jacka, F. N., et al. (2009). Association between magnesium intake and depression and anxiety in community-dwelling adults: the Hordaland Health Study. The Australian and New Zealand Journal of Psychiatry, 43(1).

62 Banki, C. M., et al. (1985). Cerebrospinal fluid magnesium and calcium related to amine metabolites, diagnosis, and suicide attempts. Biological Psychiatry, 20(2).

63 Levine, J., et al. (1999). High serum and cerebrospinal fluid Ca/Mg ratio in recently hospitalized acutely depressed patients. Neuropsychobiology, 39.

64 Ibid.

65 Whittle, N., et al. (2011). Changes in brain protein expression are linked to magnesium restriction-induced depression-like behavior. Amino Acids, 40.

66 Barchas, J., et al. (1963). Brain amines: Response to physiological stress. Biochemical Pharmacology, 12.

67 Carboni, L., et al. (2006). Proteomic analysis of rat hippocampus and frontal cortex after chronic treatment with fluoxetine or putative novel antidepressants: CRF1 and NK1 receptor antagonists. Eur Neuropsychopharmacolog., 16.

68 Beasley, C. L., et al. (2006). Proteomic analysis of the anterior cingulate cortex in the major psychiatric disorders: evidence for disease-associated changes. Proteomics, 6.

69 Iosifescu, D. V., et al. (2008). Brain bioenergetics and response to triiodothyronine augmentation in major depressive disorder. Biological Psychiatry,63.

70 Walton, J., et al. (2013). Neuronal nitric oxide synthase and NADPH oxidase interact to affect cognitive, affective, and social behaviors in mice. Behavioural Brain Research, 256.

71 Mak, I. T., et al. (1995). NO inhibition attenuates Mg-deficiency-induced oxidative injury in vivo. FASEB J, 9.

72 Barragan-Rodriguez, L., et al. (2008). Efficacy and safety of oral magnesium supplementation in the treatment of depression in the elderly with type 2 diabetes: a randomized, equivalent trial. Magnesium Research, 21.

73 Walker, A., et al. (2009). Magnesium Supplementation Alleviates Premenstrual Symptoms of Fluid Retention. Journal of Women's Health, 7.

74 Facchinetti, F., et al. (1991). Oral magnesium successfully relieves premenstrual mood changes. Obstetrics& Gynecology, 78.

Bibliography

75 Facchinetti, F., et al. (2005). Magnesium prophylaxis of menstrual migraine: effects on intracellular magnesium. Headache: The Journal of Head and Face Pain, 5.

76 Quaranta, S., et al. (2007). Pilot study of the efficacy and safety of a modified-release magnesium 250 mg tablet for the treatment of premenstrual syndrome. Clinical Drug Investigation, 27.

77 Bottiglieri, T. (2005). Homocysteine and folate metabolism in depression. Progress in Neuro-Psychopharmacology and Biological Psychiatry, 29.

78 Ibid

79 Coppen, A., et al. (2005). Treatment of depression: time to consider folic acid and vitamin B12. Journal of Psychopharmacology, 19

80 Penninx, B. W., et al. (2000). Vitamin B(12) deficiency and depression in physically disabled older women; epidemiologic evidence from the Women's Health and Aging Study. The American Journal of Psychiatry, 157.

81 Syed, E. U., et al. (2013). Vitamin B12 supplementation in treating major depressive disorder: a randomized controlled trial. The Open Neurology Journal.

82 Alpert, J. E., et al. (2000). Nutrition and depression: focus on folate. Nutrition, 16.

83 Bjelland, I., et al. (2003). Folate, vitamin B12, homocysteine and the MTHFR 677C-T polymorphism in anxiety and depression: the Hordaland homocysteine study. Archives of General Psychiatry, 6.

84 Rosche, J., et al. (2003). Low serum folate levels as a risk factor for depressive mood in patients with chronic epilepsy. The Journal of Neuropsychiatry and Clinical Neurosciences, 15.

85 Alpert, J. E., et al. (2000). Nutrition and depression: focus on folate. Nutrition, 16.

86 Papakostas, G., et al. (2012). L-methylfolate as adjunctive therapy for SSRI-resistant major depression: results of two randomized, double-blind, parallel-sequential trials. American Journal of Psychiatry, 169(12).

87 Owen, A. J. (2005). Low plasma vitamin E levels in major depression: diet or disease? European Journal of Clinical Nutrition, 59.

88 Maes, M. et al. (2000). Lower serum vitamin E concentrations in major depression. Another marker of lowered antioxidant defenses in that illness. Journal of Affective Disorders 58(3).

89 Tiemeier, H., et al. (2002). Vitamin E and depressive symptoms are not related. The Rotterdam Study. Journal of Affective Disorders, 72(1).

90 Finley, J & Penland, J. (1998). Adequacy or deprivation of dietary selenium in healthy men: Clinical and psychological findings. The Journal of Trace Elements in Experimental Medicine.
91 Benton, D. & Cook, R. (1991). The impact of selenium supplementation on mood. Biological Psychiatry, 29 (11).

92 Lambert, N. M., et al. (2011). Gratitude and depressive symptoms: the role of positive reframing and positive emotion. Cognition & Emotion, 26(4).

Bibliography

93 Wood, A., et al. (2008). The role of gratitude in the development of social support, stress, and depression: Two longitudinal studies. Journal of Research in Personality, 42, 4.

94 Lambert, N. M., et al. (2011). Gratitude and depressive symptoms: the role of positive reframing and positive emotion. Cognition & Emotion, 26(4).

95   Http://www.dailymail.co.uk/health/article-2280869/Feeling-blue-Then-try-tango-Scientists-claim-dance-helps-rid-depression-anxiety-stress.html#ixzz4AM4Mzzk4

42747790R00054

Made in the USA
San Bernardino, CA
08 December 2016